CONTENTS

Mastering Spanish for Healthcare Professionals   1

COPYRIGHTS   2

Author: OA PUBLICATIONS   3

Chapter 1   8

Chapter 2   15

Chapter 3   26

Chapter 4   32

Chapter 5   38

Chapter 6   47

MASTERING SPANISH FOR HEALTHCARE PROFESSIONALS

OBGYN Edition

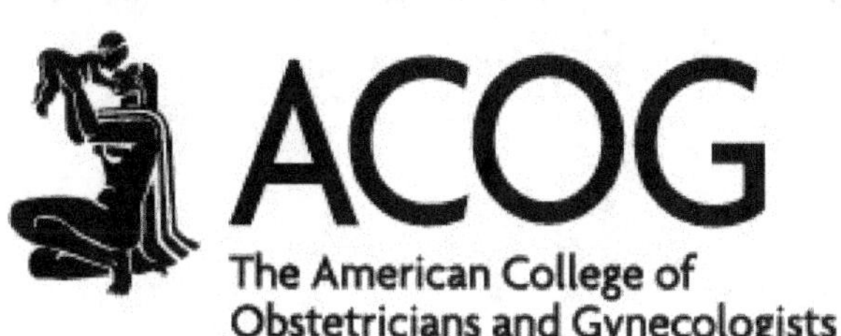

COPYRIGHTS

AUTHOR: OA PUBLICATIONS

Introduction:

In the dynamic world of healthcare, effective communication plays a pivotal role in providing exceptional patient care. As a healthcare professional, being able to communicate fluently and confidently with patients can make all the difference. "Mastering Spanish for Healthcare Professionals: OBGYN Edition" is a comprehensive guide designed to empower healthcare practitioners in the obstetrics and gynecology field with the language skills they need to navigate patient interactions seamlessly.

This specialized edition of "Mastering Spanish for Healthcare Professionals" is tailored for obstetricians and gynecologists, as well as other healthcare providers who interact with Spanish-speaking patients in women's health. In this book, you'll find a carefully curated collection of common phrases and essential medical vocabulary, specifically focused on the unique challenges and scenarios encountered in obstetrics and gynecology. Whether you're conducting examinations, discussing treatment options, or providing prenatal care, this book equips you with the language tools to effectively connect with your patients and provide the best possible care.

Our goal is to help you bridge the language barrier and enhance your patient relationships. With real-world examples, practical dialogues, and insightful tips, "Mastering Spanish for Healthcare Professionals: OBGYN Edition" is not just a language resource; it's a valuable companion that empowers you to confidently communicate, build trust, and ultimately contribute to better patient outcomes.

In the following chapters, we'll explore a range of scenarios and conversations that are central to your role in women's health. From addressing pregnancy-related concerns to explaining medical procedures, this book covers the spectrum of interactions you'll encounter in your practice. Each chapter provides you with the tools to engage in meaningful conversations and ensure that your patients receive the highest quality of care.

Whether you're a seasoned practitioner or just starting your journey in the world of obstetrics and gynecology, "Mastering Spanish for Healthcare Professionals: OBGYN Edition" is your roadmap to effective communication and professional excellence. Let's embark on this journey together, as we equip you with the language skills that will make a positive impact on the lives of your patients.

Greetings and Basic Phrases:

Hello / Hi - Hola
Good morning - Buenos días
Good afternoon - Buenas tardes
Good evening - Buenas noches
How are you? - ¿Cómo está usted?
I am a doctor - Soy médico
How can I help you? - ¿En qué puedo ayudarle?
What is the problem? - ¿Cuál es el problema?
Where does it hurt? - ¿Dónde le duele?
Are you in pain? - ¿Siente dolor?
Do you understand? - ¿Entiende?
Yes - Sí
No - No
Thank you - Gracias
You're welcome - De nada
Please - Por favor
Excuse me / Sorry - Perdón / Disculpe

Medical Vocabulary:

Patient - Paciente
Doctor - Médico
Nurse - Enfermero/a
Hospital - Hospital
Clinic - Clínica
Appointment - Cita
Prescription – Receta médica
Medicine - Medicina
Pain - Dolor
Fever - Fiebre
Cold - Resfriado
Cough - Tos
Headache - Dolor de cabeza
Stomachache - Dolor de estómago
Allergy - Alergia
Breathing difficulty - Dificultad para respirar
Blood pressure - Presión arterial
Heart - Corazón
Lungs - Pulmones
X-ray - Radiografía
Test - Examen
Surgery - Cirugía

Useful Phrases for Medical Situations:

I need to examine you - Necesito examinarlo/a
Take a deep breath - Respire profundo
Show me where it hurts - Muéstreme dónde le duele
Lie down, please - Acuéstese, por favor
Can you describe the pain? - ¿Puede describir el dolor?
I will give you a prescription - Le daré una receta médico
You should take this medicine - Debe tomar esta medicina
We need to run some tests - Necesitamos hacer algunos exámenes
You need surgery - Necesita cirugía
It's important to follow the treatment - Es importante seguir el tratamiento
Remember, practice is key when learning a new language. Start by incorporating these phrases into your interactions with Spanish-speaking patients. Additionally, consider using language learning apps, online courses, or hiring a tutor to further improve your Spanish skills. As you progress, you can expand your vocabulary and improve your conversational abilities. Good luck!

CHAPTER 1

Building a rapport with the patient

Building rapport is like laying the foundation for effective communication and meaningful connections. Whether you're a doctor, teacher, or anyone engaging with others, creating a genuine bond is essential. This connection isn't just a social nicety; it's a catalyst for trust, understanding, and successful outcomes.

- To say "My name is Doctor 'so and so'" in Spanish, you would say:

"Mi nombre es Doctor 'fulano de tal'."

Here's the breakdown of the sentence:
"Mi" means "My."
"Nombre" means "name."
"Es" means "is."
"Doctor" is used as is.
"'fulano de tal'" stands for the specific name you want to use.

- To say "I am the doctor in the clinic today" in Spanish, you would say:

"Soy el médico en la clínica hoy."

Here's the breakdown of the sentence:
"Soy" means "I am."
"el médico" means "the doctor" (masculine form).

"en la clínica" means "in the clinic."
"hoy" means "today."

- To say "I am the on-call doctor today" in Spanish, you would say:

<u>"Soy el médico de guardia hoy."</u>

Here's the breakdown of the sentence:
"Soy" means "I am."
"el médico" means" the doctor."
"de guardia" means "on-call."
"hoy" means "today."

- To say "How are you feeling?" in Spanish, you would say:

<u>"¿Cómo te sientes?"</u>

Here's the breakdown of the sentence:
"¿Cómo" means "How."
"te" is the informal second person singular pronoun "you."
"sientes" is the second person singular form of the verb "sentir," which means "to feel."

- To say "Have we met before?" in Spanish, you would say:

<u>"¿Nos hemos conocido antes?"</u>

Here's the breakdown of the sentence:
"¿Nos" means "We."
"hemos" is the first person plural form of the verb "haber," which

means "to have" in this context.

"conocido" is the past participle of the verb "conocer," which means "to meet" or "to know."

"antes" means "before."

- To say "I don't believe we have met" in Spanish, you would say:

<u>"No creo que nos hayamos conocido."</u>

Here's the breakdown of the sentence:

"No" means "Not" or "No."

"creo" means "I believe." It is the first-person singular form of the verb "creer."

"que" means "that."

"nos" means "we" (referring to ourselves).

"hayamos conocido" is the first person plural form of the verb "haber" (to have) combined with the past participle "conocido" (met) of the verb "conocer" (to meet).

- To say "Do you remember me?" in Spanish, you would say:

<u>"¿Te acuerdas de mí?"</u>

Here's the breakdown of the sentence:

"¿Te" is the informal second person singular pronoun "you."

"acuerdas" is the second person singular form of the verb "acordar," which means "to remember" or "to recall."

"de mí" means "of me."

-    To say "Who is your regular doctor?" in Spanish, you would say:

<u>"¿Quién es su médico regular?"</u>

Here's the breakdown of the sentence:
"¿Quién" means "Who."
"es" is the third person singular form of the verb "ser," which means "to be" in this context. "su" means "your" (formal).
"médico" means "doctor."
"regular" means "regular."

To say "I would like to ask you a few questions" in Spanish, you say:

<u>"Me gustaría hacerte algunas preguntas."</u>

Here's the breakdown of the sentence:
"Me gustaría" means "I would like."
"hacerte" means "to ask you" (using the pronoun "te" for "you").
"algunas" means "a few or some"
"preguntas" means "questions."

Extra:

1- In Spanish, sometimes <u>adjectives come after nouns</u>, which is a bit different from English. This happens for a few reasons:

Emphasis and Specific Details:
Placing adjectives after nouns makes them stand out more and gives specific information.
Example:
Instead of saying "a big house," you say "una casa grande."

Feelings and Qualities:
When talking about feelings or qualities, Spanish often puts adjectives after nouns.
Example:
Instead of saying "a happy moment," you say "un momento feliz."

Inherent Characteristics:
Certain adjectives naturally come after nouns in Spanish.
Example:
Instead of saying "a red flower," you say "una flor roja."

2- <u>"Haber" and "Tener"</u> are two essential verbs in Spanish, and both mean "to have", but they are used in different contexts and have distinct usage. Let's break down the differences:

Haber:

Auxiliary Verb for Perfect Tesnses: "Haber" is primarily used as an auxiliary verb to form perfect tenses in Spanish (like the present perfect, past perfect, etc.).

Impersonal Expressions: "Haber" is used in impersonal expressions to indicate the existence of something.
Example: "Hay muchos libros en la biblioteca." (There are many books in the library.)

No Specific Subject: It's often used without specifying the subject. This is why it's commonly used in impersonal expressions.
Example: "Ha llovido mucho." (It has rained a lot.)

Tener:

Possession: "Tener" is used to indicate possession or ownership.
Example: "Tengo un perro." (I have a dog.)

Expressions of Age: It's used to express age.
Example: "Tiene veinte años." (He/She is twenty years old.)

Physical and Emotional States: It's used to express physical and emotional states.
Example: "Tengo hambre." (I am hungry.)

3- "Me gustaría" is a more formal and polite way of making a request or expressing a desire, while "me gusta" simply indicates a personal liking for something.

Here are examples to illustrate the difference between "me gustaría" and "me gusta":

"Me gustaría ir al cine mañana." (I would like to go to the movies tomorrow.)
"Me gustaría aprender a tocar la guitarra." (I would like to learn how to play the guitar.)
"Me gustaría viajar a Francia algún día." (I would like to travel to France someday.)

"Me gusta el chocolate." (I like chocolate.)
"Me gusta escuchar música en mi tiempo libre." (I like listening to

music in my free time.)
"Me gusta pasar tiempo con mi familia." (I like spending time with my family.)

CHAPTER 2

History taking:

There are frequently used phrases that you repeat consistently. Repetitively using these sentences helps you enhance your Spanish language proficiency. This practice also empowers you to combine words from various sentences to create new ones.

- To say "I would like to ask you a few questions" in Spanish, you would say:

<u>"Me gustaría hacerte algunas preguntas."</u>

Here's the breakdown of the sentence:
"Me gustaría" means "I would like."
"hacerte" means "to ask you," where "hacer" means "to ask" and "te" is the direct object pronoun for "you."
"algunas preguntas" means "a few questions."

- "How can I help you today?" in Spanish is:

<u>"¿Cómo puedo ayudarte hoy?"</u>

Here's the breakdown of the sentence:
"¿Cómo" means "How."
"puedo" means "I can" (first person singular form of the verb "poder").
"ayudarte" means "help you" (using the pronoun "te" for "you").
"hoy" means "today."

- To ask "How many times have you been pregnant?" in Spanish, you would say:

<u>"¿Cuántas veces has estado embarazada?"</u>

Here's the breakdown of the sentence:
"¿Cuántas veces?" means "How many times?"
"has" is the second person singular form of the verb "haber" (to have) in the present tense.
"estado" is the second person singular form of the verb "estar" (to be) in the present perfect tense.
"embarazada" means "pregnant."

- To ask "Have you had any problems during this pregnancy?" in Spanish, you would say:

<u>"¿Has tenido algún problema durante este embarazo?"</u>

Here's the breakdown of the sentence:
"¿Has tenido?" means "Have you had?" where "has" is the second person singular form of the verb "haber" (to have) in the present tense, and "tenido" is the past participle of "tener."
"algún" means "any."
"problema" means " problem."
"durante" means "during. "
"este" means "this. "
"embarazo" means "pregnancy."

Now you understand that:

Embarazo means pregnancy
Embarazada means pregnant

- To ask "How many weeks are you?" in Spanish, you would say:

"¿Cuántas semanas tienes?"

Here's the breakdown of the sentence:
"¿Cuántas" means "how many."
"semanas?" means " weeks?"
"tienes" is the second person singular form of the verb "tener" (to have) in the present tense.

- To ask "Have you had an ultrasound during this pregnancy?" in Spanish, you would say:

"¿Has tenido un ultrasonido durante este embarazo?"

Here's the breakdown of the sentence:
"¿Has tenido?" means "Have you had?" where "has" is the second person singular form of the verb "haber" (to have) in the present tense, and "tenido" is the past participle of "tener."
"ultrasonido" means "an ultrasound."
"durante este embarazo" means "during this pregnancy."

- To ask "Have you had all your blood tests during this

pregnancy?" in Spanish, you would say:

"¿Has tenido todos tus análisis de sangre durante este embarazo?"

Here's the breakdown of the sentence:
"¿Has tenido?" means "Have you had?"
"todos" means "all, all of. "
"tus" means "your."
"análisis de sangre" means "all your blood tests."
"durante este embarazo" means "during this pregnancy."

- To ask "Did you pass your diabetes test?" in Spanish, you would say:

"¿Pasaste tu prueba de diabetes?"

Here's the breakdown of the sentence:
"¿Pasaste?" means "Did you pass?" where "pasaste" is the second person singular form of the verb "pasar" (to pass) in the past tense.
"tu prueba de diabetes" means "your diabetes test."

Now you understand that tu means yours in a singular form, and tus means yours in a plural form.

- To ask "Do you have any pain anywhere?" in Spanish, you would say:

"¿Tiene algún dolor en alguna parte?"

Here's the breakdown of the sentence:
"¿Tiene?" means "Do you have?" where "tiene" is the third person

singular form of the verb "tener" (to have) in the present tense.
"algún dolor" means "any pain."
"en alguna parte" means "anywhere."

We have used the word "Algún" in multiple places. So, this is a good place to review it. It's equivalent to "some" or "any" in English. For example:

- "Algún" (masculine singular):
"Algún libro" (Some book)
"¿Tienes algún problema?" (Do you have any problem?)
- "Alguna" (feminine singular):
"Alguna amiga" (Some friend - female)
"¿Tienes alguna pregunta?" (Do you have any question?)
- "Algunas" (feminine plural):
"Algunas flores" (Some flowers)
"¿Tienes algunas dudas?" (Do you have any concerns?)

In summary:
"Algún" is used with masculine singular nouns.
"Alguna" is used with feminine singular nouns.
"Algunas" is used with feminine plural nouns.
All three forms convey the idea of "some" or "any," and they agree with the gender and number of the nouns they modify.

"Hemos" and "hayamos" are both forms of the verb "haber," but they are used in different tenses and moods:

"Hemos" is the first-person plural form of the present perfect tense of "haber."
It's used when talking about actions that have been completed in the past but have relevance to the present.

Example: "Hemos comido" means "We have eaten."

"Hayamos" is the first person plural form of the present subjunctive tense of "haber."
It's used in situations where there is uncertainty, doubt, desire, or suggestions.
Example: "Espero que hayamos llegado a tiempo" means "I hope that we have arrived on time."

In summary, "hemos" is used in the present perfect tense to indicate completed actions with relevance to the present, while "hayamos" is used in the present subjunctive tense for situations involving uncertainty, doubt, desire, or suggestions.

-       To say "Where is your pain?" in Spanish, you would say:

"¿Dónde está tu dolor?"

Here's the breakdown of the sentence:
"¿Dónde " means "where."
"está" is the third person singular form of the verb "estar" (to be) in the present tense.
"tu dolor" means "your pain."

-       To say "How long have you had this pain?" in Spanish, you would say:

"¿Cuánto tiempo ha tenido este dolor?"

Here's the breakdown of the sentence:
"¿Cuánto ctiempo" means "how long,"
"has tenido" means "have you had."
"este dolor" means "this pain."

- Have you noticed we used "Ha" instead of "Has"? let's dive a little bit deeper.

"Ha" and "has" are both forms of the verb "haber" (to have) in Spanish, but they are conjugated differently based on the subject pronoun and the tense being used.

Let's break down the differences:

"Ha tenido" is the third person singular form of the present perfect tense.

It is used with the subject pronoun "él," "ella," or "usted" (he, she, or you formal).
It translates to "he has had," "she has had," or "you have had" in English.
Example: "Él ha tenido mucho éxito en su carrera." (He has had a lot of success in his career.)

"Has tenido" is the second person singular form of the present perfect tense.

It is used with the subject pronoun "tú" (you informal singular).
It translates to "you have had" in English.
Example: "¿Has tenido alguna experiencia similar antes?" (Have you had a similar experience before?)

- To say "Does anything make it better or worse?" in Spanish, you would say:

"<u>¿Hay algo que lo haga mejorar o empeorar?</u>"

Here's the breakdown of the sentence:
"¿Hay" means "is there? Or there is."
"algo" means "something."
" que" means "that."
"lo" means "it."
"haga?" is the third person singular form of the verb "hacer" (to make/do) in the present subjunctive tense.
"mejorar" means "better."
"empeorar" means "worse."

- To say "Do you have any bleeding?" in Spanish, you would say:

"<u>¿Tiene algún sangrado?</u>"

Here's the breakdown of the sentence:
"¿Tiene?" means "Do you have?" where "tiene" is the third person singular form of the verb "tener" (to have) in the present tense.
"algún sangrado" means "any bleeding."

- To say "How much blood have you lost?" in Spanish, you would say:

"<u>¿Cuánta sangre has perdido?</u>"

Here's the breakdown of the sentence:
"¿Cuánta" means "how much."
"sangre?" means "blood."
"has" was explained previously
"perdido" is the second person singular form of the verb "perder" (to lose) in the present perfect tense.

-    To say "Has the bleeding stopped?" in Spanish, you would say:

"¿Ha parado el sangrado?"

Here's the breakdown of the sentence:
"ha" is the third person singular form of the verb "haber" (to have) in the present tense. "parado" is the past participle of the verb "parar" (to stop).
"el sangrado" means "the bleeding."

-    To say "Do you have any medical problem?" in Spanish, you would say:

"¿Tiene algún problema médico?"

Here's the breakdown of the sentence:
"¿Tiene?" means "Do you have?" where "tiene" is the third person singular form of the verb "tener" (to have) in the present tense.
"algún " means " any"
"problema" means "problem"
"médico" means "medical"

To say "Have you had any surgeries?" in Spanish, you would say:

"¿Ha tenido alguna cirugía?"

Here's the breakdown of the sentence:
"¿Ha tenido?" means "Have you had?" where "ha" is the third person singular form of the verb "haber" (to have) in the present tense.
"tenido" is the past participle of the verb "tener" (to have).
"alguna cirugía" means "any surgeries."

- To say "Are you on any regular medications?" in Spanish, you would say:

<u>"¿Está tomando algún medicamento regular?"</u>

Here's the breakdown of the sentence:
"¿Está tomando?" means "Are you taking?" where "está" is the third person singular form of the verb "estar" (to be) in the present tense, and "tomando" is the present participle of the verb "tomar" (to take).
"algún medicamento regular" means "any regular medications."

- To say "Are you allergic to anything?" in Spanish, you would say:

<u>"¿Es alérgico/a a algo?"</u>

Here's the breakdown of the sentence:
"¿Es alérgico/a?" means "Are you allergic?" where "es" is the third person singular form of the verb "ser" (to be) in the present tense, and "alérgico/a" means "allergic."
"a" means "to."
"algo" means "anything."

- To say "Do you smoke, drink alcohol, or take any drugs?" in Spanish, you would say:

<u>"¿Fuma, bebe alcohol o toma drogas?"</u>

Fuma: This is the third person singular form of the verb "fumar," which means "to smoke."
Bebe:This is the third person singular form of the verb "beber," which means "to drink."

"alcohol" means "alcohol"
"o" This is the conjunction "or" in Spanish, used to connect alternatives.
"toma" This is the third person singular form of the verb "tomar," which means "to take" or "to consume."
"drogas" means "drugs."

- To say "Do you have any family history of medical problems?" in Spanish, you would say:

<u>"¿Tiene antecedentes familiares de problemas médicos?"</u>

Here's the breakdown of the sentence:
"¿Tiene?" means "Do you have?" where "tiene" is the third person singular form of the verb "tener" (to have) in the present tense.
"antecedentes" means "history."
"familiares" means "family."
"de problemas médicos" means "of medical problems."

CHAPTER 3

Examination:

- To say "I would like to examine you" in Spanish, you would say:

"Me gustaría examinarlo/a."

Here's the breakdown of the sentence:
"Me gustaría" means "I would like."
"examinarlo/a" means "to examine you," where "lo" or "la" is added depending on the gender of the person you're addressing.

- To say "I would like to examine your abdomen" in Spanish, you would say:

"Me gustaría examinarle el abdomen."

Here's the breakdown of the sentence:
"Me gustaría" means "I would like."
"examinarle" means "to examine you," where "le" is used as a formal way to address the person.
"el abdomen" means "the abdomen."

- To say "I would like to check your cervix" in Spanish, you would say:

"Me gustaría revisar su cuello uterino."

Here's the breakdown of the sentence:

"Me gustaría" means "I would like."
"revisar" means "to check."
"su" means "your."
"cuello uterino" means "cervix."

- To say "I would like to do an ultrasound scan" in Spanish, you would say:

"Me gustaría hacer un ultrasonido."

Here's the breakdown of the sentence:
"Me gustaría" means "I would like."
"hacer" means "to do."
"un ultrasonido" means "an ultrasound scan."

- To say "I would like to scan your baby" in Spanish, you would say:

"Me gustaría hacer un ultrasonido a su bebé."

Here's the breakdown of the sentence:
"Me gustaría" means "I would like."
"hacer" means "to do."
"un ultrasonido" means "an ultrasound scan."
"a su bebé" means "to your baby."

- To say "I would like to examine you" in Spanish, you would say:

"Me gustaría examinarte."

Here's the breakdown of the sentence:
"Me gustaría" means "I would like."
"examinarte" means "to examine you," where "examinar" means

"to examine" and "te" is the direct object pronoun for "you."

Here are the translations for "I would like to examine your [body part]" in Spanish:
I would like to examine your neck: "Me gustaría examinarle el cuello."
I would like to examine your breast: "Me gustaría examinarle el ceno."
I would like to examine your chest: "Me gustaría examinarle el ceno."
I would like to examine your abdomen: "Me gustaría examinarle el abdomen."
In these sentences, "Me gustaría examinarle" means "I would like to examine you," and the specific body part is indicated by "el cuello" (neck), "el ceno/pecho" (breast/chest), or "el abdomen" (abdomen). "Le" is used as a formal way to address the patient.

- To say "I would like to listen to your heart and lungs" in Spanish, you would say:

"Me gustaría escuchar su corazón y pulmones."

Here's the breakdown of the sentence:
"Me gustaría" means "I would like."
"escuchar" means "to listen."
"su corazón y pulmones" means "your heart and lungs," where "su" is used as a formal way to address the patient.

- To say "I would like to do a vaginal examination" in Spanish, you would say:

"Me gustaría hacer un examen vaginal."

Here's the breakdown of the sentence:

"Me gustaría" means "I would like."
"hacer" means "to do."
"un examen vaginal" means "a vaginal examination."
So, the phrase translates to "I would like to do a vaginal examination." As always, it's important to communicate such procedures clearly and with sensitivity, obtaining informed consent from the patient.

- To say "I will use a speculum to look at the cervix" in Spanish, you would say:

"Voy a usar un espéculo para observar el cuello uterino."

Here's the breakdown of the sentence:
"Voy a usar" means "I will use."
"un espéculo" means "a speculum," which is used in medical examinations.
"para" means "for or to"
"observar" means "to look" or "to observe."
"el cuello uterino" means "the cervix."

- To say "I would like to take swabs/pap smear" in Spanish, you would say:

"Me gustaría tomar muestras/realizar un Papanicolaou."

Here's the breakdown of the sentence:
"Me gustaría" means "I would like."
"tomar muestras" means "to take samples," referring to swabs.
"realizar" means "to perform"
"un Papanicolaou" means "a Pap smear,"

- To say "The swabs are to detect any infection" in Spanish, you would say:

<u>"Las muestras son para detectar cualquier infección."</u>

Here's the breakdown of the sentence:
"Las muestras" means "The samples" or "The swabs."
"son" means "are"
"para" means "for."
"detectar" means "detect"
"cualquier infección" means "detect any infection."

- To say "The Pap smear is to detect any abnormal cells that can turn into cancer without treatment" in Spanish, you would say:

<u>"El Papanicolaou es para detectar células anormales que pueden convertirse en cáncer sin tratamiento."</u>

Here's the breakdown of the sentence:
"El Papanicolaou" refers to the "Pap smear" test.
"es para" means "is for."
"detectar células anormales" means "detect abnormal cells."
"que" means "that"
"pueden" means "can"
"convertirse" means "convert"
"en cáncer" means "to cancer"

"sin" means "without"
"tratamiento" means "treatment."

CHAPTER 4
Labor and Delivery:

- To say "I would like to rupture your membranes" in Spanish, you would say:

<u>"Me gustaría romper sus membranas."</u>

Here's the breakdown of the sentence:
"Me gustaría" means "I would like."
"romper" means "to rupture" or "to break."
"sus membranas" means "your membranes," where "sus" is used to indicate the formal address.

- To say "I would like to insert internal monitors to monitor the contractions and the baby's heartbeat" in Spanish, you would say:

<u>"Me gustaría colocar monitores internos para monitorear las contracciones y el latido del corazón del bebé."</u>

Here's the breakdown of the sentence:
"Me gustaría" means "I would like."
"colocar" means "to place" or "to insert."
"monitores internos" means "internal monitors."
"para" means "to or for. "
"<u>monitorear</u>" means "monitor."
"las contracciones" means "the contractions."
"y" means "and."
" el latido del corazón" means "heartbeat."

"del bebé" means "of the baby."

- To say "You are 5 cm dilated" in Spanish, you would say:

<u>"Está dilatada 5 centímetros."</u>

Here's the breakdown of the sentence:
"Está" means "You are" (formal) where "está" is the third person singular form of the verb "estar" (to be) in the present tense.
"dilatada" means "dilated" (referring to the cervix being dilated).
"5 centímetros" means "5 centimeters."

- To say "You are completely dilated" in Spanish, you would say:

<u>"Está completamente dilatada."</u>

Here's the breakdown of the sentence:
"Está" means "You are" (formal) where "está" is the third person singular form of the verb "estar" (to be) in the present tense.
"completamente dilatada" means "completely dilated."

- To say "We can start pushing" in Spanish, you would say:

<u>"Podemos empezar a empujar."</u>

Here's the breakdown of the sentence:
"Podemos" means "We can."
"empezar a" means "to start."
"empujar" means "pushing."

- To say "The baby's heartbeat is normal" in Spanish, you would say:

<u>"El latido del corazón del bebé es normal."</u>

Here's the breakdown of the sentence:
"El latido del corazón del bebé" means "The baby's heartbeat."
"es normal" means "is normal."

- To say "The baby's heartbeat is abnormal" in Spanish, you would say:

<u>"El latido del corazón del bebé es anormal."</u>

Here's the breakdown of the sentence:
"El latido del corazón del bebé" means "The baby's heartbeat."
"es anormal" means "is abnormal."

- To say "I am concerned about the baby's heartbeat" in Spanish, you would say:

<u>"Me preocupa el latido del corazón del bebé."</u>

Here's the breakdown of the sentence:
"Me preocupa" means "I am concerned."
"el latido del corazón del bebé" means "the baby's heartbeat."

- To say "I would like to perform a cesarean section" in Spanish, you would say:

<u>"Me gustaría realizar una cesárea."</u>

Here's the breakdown of the sentence:
"Me gustaría" means "I would like."
"realizar" means "to perform."
"una cesárea" means "a cesarean section."

- To say "I would like to perform a forceps delivery" in Spanish, you would say:

<u>"Me gustaría realizar un parto con fórceps."</u>

Here's the breakdown of the sentence:
"Me gustaría" means "I would like."
"realizar" means "to perform."
"un parto con fórceps" means "a forceps delivery."

- To say "I would like to perform a vacuum delivery" in Spanish, you would say:

<u>"Me gustaría realizar un parto con ventosa."</u>

Here's the breakdown of the sentence:
"Me gustaría" means "I would like."
"realizar" means "to perform."
"un parto con ventosa" means "a vacuum delivery."

To say "You have a small vaginal tear" in Spanish:

<u>"Tienes un pequeño desgarro vaginal."</u>

Here's the breakdown of the sentence:
"Tienes" means "You have" (second person singular of the verb "tener").
"un" means "a" or "an."
"pequeño" means "small."
"desgarro" means "tear" or "laceration."
"vaginal" means "vaginal."

To say "I will suture the tear" in Spanish:

<u>"Voy a suturar el desgarro."</u>

Here's the breakdown of the sentence:
"Voy a" means "I will" (first person singular of the verb "ir" in future tense, plus "a" which indicates future action).
"suturar" means "to suture."
"el" means "the" (masculine singular article).
"desgarro" means "tear."

To say "If you have pain, tell me so that I can give you local anesthesia" in Spanish:

"Si tienes dolor, avísame para que pueda administrarte anestesia local."

Here's the breakdown of the sentence:
"Si" means "If."
"tienes" means "you have" (second person singular of the verb "tener").
"dolor" means "pain."
"avísame" means "tell me" (imperative form of the verb "avisar").
"para que" means "so that."
"pueda" means "I can" (first person singular of the verb "poder" in subjunctive form).
"administrarte" means "to administer to you."
"anestesia local" means "local anesthesia."

CHAPTER 5

Consent:

- To say "The risk of this procedure is a small bruise, injury to the baby, and injury to the vagina and the rectum" in Spanish, you would say:

<u>"El riesgo de este procedimiento es un pequeño moretón, lesiones al bebé y lesiones en la vagina y el recto."</u>

Here's the breakdown of the sentence:
"El riesgo" means "the risk"
"de este" means "of this"
"procedimiento" means "procedure."
"un pequeño" means "a small
"moretón" means "bruise."
"lesiones al bebé" means "injury to the baby."
"lesiones en la vagina y el recto" means "injury to the vagina and the rectum."

- To say "The risk of this procedure is bleeding, infection, injury to the bladder or the bowel, risk of anesthesia, and risk of blood clots in the legs" in Spanish, you would say:

<u>"El riesgo de este procedimiento incluye sangrado, infección, lesiones en la vejiga o el intestino, riesgo de anestesia y riesgo de coágulos sanguíneos en las piernas."</u>

Here's the breakdown of the sentence:

"El riesgo de este procedimiento incluye" means "The risk of this procedure includes."
"sangrado" means "bleeding."
"infección" means "infection."
"lesiones en la vejiga o el intestino" means "injury to the bladder or the bowel."
"riesgo de anestesia" means "risk of anesthesia."
"riesgo de coágulos sanguíneos" means "risk of blood clots"
"en las piernas" means "in the legs."

- To say "Do you understand everything?" in Spanish, you would say:

"¿Entiendes todo?"

Here's the breakdown of the sentence:
"¿Entiendes?" means "Do you understand?" where "entiendes" is the second person singular form of the verb "entender" (to understand) in the present tense.
"todo" means "everything."

- To say "Do you have any questions?" in Spanish, you would say:

"¿Tiene alguna pregunta?"

Here's the breakdown of the sentence:
"¿Tiene?" means "Do you have?" where "tiene" is the third person singular form of the verb "tener" (to have) in the present tense.
"alguna pregunta" means "any questions."

- To say "Can you sign here?" in Spanish, you would say:

"¿Puede firmar aquí?"

Here's the breakdown of the sentence:
"¿Puede?" means "Can you?" where "puede" is the third person singular form of the verb "poder" (to be able to) in the present tense.
"firmar" means "to sign."
"aquí" means "here."

- To say "Is anybody with you?" in Spanish, you would say:

<u>"¿Hay alguien contigo?"</u>

Here's the breakdown of the sentence:
"¿Hay" means "there is" or "there are,"
"alguien" means "anybody."
"contigo" means "with you."

"Ser" (to be) is used to describe inherent or permanent characteristics, identity, origin, professions, and general qualities.

"Soy médico." (I am a doctor.) - Describing a profession.
"Ella es inteligente." (She is intelligent.) - Inherent quality.
"Somos de México." (We are from Mexico.) - Origin.
"Ellos son mis amigos." (They are my friends.) - Identity.

"Estar" (to be) is used to describe temporary states, emotions, locations, and conditions that can change.

"Estoy cansado/a." (I am tired.) - Temporary state.
"Ella está feliz." (She is happy.) - Emotional state.
"Estamos en casa." (We are at home.) - Location.
"La comida está caliente." (The food is hot.) - Condition that can change.

- To say "I would like to take a biopsy from the lining of the uterus" in Spanish, you would say:

<u>"Me gustaría tomar una biopsia del revestimiento del útero."</u>

Here's the breakdown of the sentence:
"Me gustaría" means "I would like."
"tomar una biopsia" means "to take a biopsy."
"del revestimiento" means "from the lining"
"del útero" means "of the uterus."

- To say "The main goal is to rule out cancer" in Spanish, you would say:

<u>"El objetivo principal es descartar el cáncer."</u>

Here's the breakdown of the sentence:
"El objetivo" means "the goal."
"principal" means "main"
"es descartar" means "is to rule out."
"el cáncer" means "cancer."

- To say "The risk of this procedure is pain, bleeding, infection, perforation of the uterus, and drop in blood pressure" in Spanish, you would say:

"El riesgo de este procedimiento incluye dolor, sangrado, infección, perforación del útero y disminución de la presión arterial."

Here's the breakdown of the sentence:
"El riesgo de este procedimiento incluye" means "The risk of this procedure includes."
"dolor" means "pain."
"sangrado" means "bleeding."
"infección" means "infection."
"perforación del útero" means "perforation of the uterus."
"disminución de la presión arterial" means "drop in blood pressure."

- To say "The main goal is to rule out cancer" in Spanish, you would say:

"El objetivo principal es descartar el cáncer."

Here's the breakdown of the sentence:
"El objetivo principal" means "The main goal."
"es descartar" means "is to rule out."
"el cáncer" means "cancer."

So, the phrase translates to "The main goal is to rule out cancer." This statement clarifies the primary objective of the procedure.

-    To say "The biopsy will be sent for histological examination" in Spanish, you would say:

"La biopsia será enviada para examen histológico."

Here's the breakdown of the sentence:
"La biopsia" means "The biopsy."
"será enviada" means "will be sent."
"para examen histológico" means "for histological examination."

-    To say "It will take five to seven days to get the results back" in Spanish, you would say:

"Tomará de cinco a siete días para obtener los resultados."

Here's the breakdown of the sentence:
"Tomará" means "It will take."
"de cinco a siete días" means "five to seven days."
"obtener los resultados" means "to get the results."

-    To say "I will give you a follow-up appointment to discuss the results" in Spanish,

"Le daré una cita de seguimiento para hablar sobre los resultados."

Here's the breakdown of the sentence:
"Le daré" means "I will give you," where "le" is the formal pronoun

for "you."
"una cita" means "an appointment
"de seguimiento" means "follow-up."
"para hablar sobre" means "to discuss or talk about."
"los resultados" means "the results.

- To say "I would like to book you for a hysteroscopy" in Spanish, you would say:

"Me gustaría programarle una histeroscopia."

Here's the breakdown of the sentence:
"Me gustaría" means "I would like."
"programarle" means "to book you," where "programarle" is the formal way to say "book you" or "schedule for you."
"una histeroscopia" means "a hysteroscopy."

- To say "It involves putting a camera inside the uterus while you're under general anesthesia" in Spanish, you would say:

"Consiste en introducir una cámara dentro del útero mientras está bajo anestesia general."

Here's the breakdown of the sentence:
"Consiste en" means "It involves" or "It consists of."
"introducir" means "putting or introduce"
"una cámara" means "a camera"
"dentro" means "inside"
"del útero" means "the uterus."
"mientras" means "while"
"está" means "you are"
"bajo" means "under"
"anestesia general" means "general anesthesia."

-       To say "The procedure takes about thirty minutes" in Spanish, you would say:

"El procedimiento dura aproximadamente treinta minutos."

Here's the breakdown of the sentence:
"El procedimiento" means "The procedure."
"dura" means "takes or lasts"
"aproximadamente" means "about"
"treinta minutos" means "thirty minutes."

-    To say "You go home on the same day" in Spanish, you would say:

"Usted regresa a casa el mismo día."

Here's the breakdown of the sentence:
"Usted regresa" means "You go back" or "You return."
"a casa" means "home"
"el mismo" means "the same"
"día" means "day."

-       To say "The risk of the procedure is bleeding, infection, injury to the cervix, perforation of the uterus, and risk of anesthesia" in Spanish, you would say:

"El riesgo del procedimiento es sangrado, infección, lesión en el cuello uterino, perforación del útero y riesgo de anestesia."

Here's the breakdown of the sentence:
"El riesgo del procedimiento es" means "The risk of the procedure is."

"sangrado" means "bleeding."
"infección" means "infection."
"lesión en el cuello uterino" means "injury to the cervix."
"perforación del útero" means "perforation of the uterus."
"riesgo de anestesia" means "risk of anesthesia."

- To say "I would like to book you for a laparoscopy" in Spanish, you would say:

<u>"Me gustaría programarle una laparoscopia."</u>

Here's the breakdown of the sentence:
"Me gustaría" means "I would like."
"programarle" means "to book you," where "programarle" is the formal way to say "book you" or "schedule for you."
"una laparoscopia" means "a laparoscopy."

- To say "The procedure is done while you're under general anesthesia" in Spanish, you would say:

<u>"El procedimiento se realiza mientras está bajo anestesia general."</u>

Here's the breakdown of the sentence:
"El procedimiento" means "The procedure."
"se realiza" means "is done" or "is performed."
"mientras está bajo anestesia general" means "while you're under general anesthesia."

CHAPTER 6

Discussing Results:

- To say "I would like to discuss the results of your blood test" in Spanish, you would say:

<u>"Me gustaría hablar sobre los resultados de su análisis de sangre."</u>

Here's the breakdown of the sentence:
"Me gustaría" means "I would like."
"hablar" means "to talk"
"sobre" means "about."
"los resultados" means "the results,"
"de su" means "of your" (formal),
"análisis de sangre" means "blood test."

- To say "I would like to discuss the result of the mammogram" in Spanish, you would say:

<u>"Me gustaría hablar sobre el resultado de la mamografía."</u>

Here's the breakdown of the sentence:
"Me gustaría" means "I would like."
"hablar sobre" means "to discuss" or "to talk about."
"el resultado" means "the result,"
"de la" means "of the,
"mamografía" means "mammogram."

- To say "I would like to discuss the result of the ultrasound" in Spanish, you would say:

<u>"Me gustaría hablar sobre el resultado de el ultrasonido."</u>

Here's the breakdown of the sentence:
"Me gustaría" means "I would like."
"hablar sobre" means "to discuss" or "to talk about."
"el resultado" means "the result,"
"<u>de el</u> ultrasonido " means "of the ultrasound."

- To say "I would like to discuss the results of the CT scan" in Spanish, you would say:

<u>"Me gustaría hablar sobre los resultados de la tomografía computarizada."</u>

Here's the breakdown of the sentence:
"Me gustaría" means "I would like."
"hablar sobre" means "to discuss" or "to talk about."
"los resultados de la tomografía computarizada" means "the results of the CT scan,"

- To say "Everything has been normal" in Spanish, you would say:

<u>"Todo ha estado normal."</u>

Here's the breakdown of the sentence:
"Todo" means "Everything."

"ha" is the third person singular form of the verb "haber" (to have) in the present tense, "estado" is the past participle of the verb "estar" (to be).
"normal" means "normal."

-     To say "Your Pap smear was abnormal" in Spanish, you would say:

<u>"Su Papanicolaou fue anormal."</u>

Here's the breakdown of the sentence:
"Su Papanicolaou" means "Your Pap smear."
"fue" means "was"
"anormal" means "abnormal."

-     To say "I would like to do a colposcopy and obtain a biopsy" in Spanish, you would say:
-

<u>"Me gustaría realizar una colposcopia y obtener una biopsia."</u>

Here's the breakdown of the sentence:
"Me gustaría" means "I would like."
"realizar" means "to perform."
"una colposcopia" means "a colposcopy."
"y obtener" means "and obtain"
"una biopsia" means "a biopsy."

-     To say "Your Pap smear showed minor abnormality" in Spanish, you would say:

<u>"Su Papanicolaou mostró una anormalidad menor."</u>

Here's the breakdown of the sentence:
"Su Papanicolaou" means "Your Pap smear."

"mostró" means "showed."
"una anormalidad" means "an abnormality"
"menor" means "minor."

- To say "The colposcope is just a magnifier" in Spanish, you would say:

"El colposcopio es simplemente un lente magnificador."

Here's the breakdown of the sentence:
"El colposcopio" means "The colposcope."
"es" means "is."
"simplemente" means "just" or "simply."
"un lente magnificador " means "a magnifier."

- To say "I will put a dye on your cervix and take a biopsy from certain areas" in Spanish, you would say:

"Voy a poner un tinte en su cuello uterino y tomar una biopsia de ciertas áreas."
Here's the breakdown of the sentence:

"Voy a" means "I will"
"poner" means "put."
"un tinte" means "a dye."
"en su cuello uterino" means "on your cervix."
"y tomar una biopsia" means "and take a biopsy."
"de ciertas áreas" means "from certain areas."

-     To say "when I take the biopsy, it might feel a pinch" in Spanish, you would say:

<u>"cuando tome la biopsia, podría sentir como un pellizco."</u>

Here's the breakdown of the sentence:
"cuando" means "when"
"tome la biopsia" means "taking the biopsy."
"podría sentir" means "might feel."
"un pellizco" means "a pinch."

-     To say "the biopsy will be sent for histological examination" in Spanish, you would say:
-

<u>"La biopsia será enviada para examen histológico."</u>

Here's the breakdown of the sentence:
"La biopsia" means "The biopsy."
"será" means "will be"
"enviada" means "sent."
"para" means "for"
"examen histológico" means "histological examination."

-     To say "it will take five to seven days to get the results back" in Spanish,

"Tomará de cinco a siete días para obtener los resultados."

Here's the breakdown of the sentence:
"Tomará" means "it will take."
"de cinco a siete días" means "five to seven days."
"obtener los resultados" means "to get the results."

- To say "I will give you an appointment to discuss the results of the biopsy" in Spanish, you would say:

"Le daré una cita para hablar sobre los resultados de la biopsia."

Here's the breakdown of the sentence:
"Le daré" means "I will give you," where "le" is the formal pronoun for "you."
"una cita" means "an appointment."
"para hablar sobre" means "to discuss or talk about."
"los resultados de la biopsia" means "the results of the biopsy."

- To say "A small amount of bleeding is to be expected" in Spanish, you would say:

"Se espera una pequeña cantidad de sangrado."

Here's the breakdown of the sentence:
"Se espera" means "is to be expected" or "is expected."
"una pequeña" means "a small"
"cantidad" means "amount"
"de sangrado" means "of bleeding."

- To say "If you have any severe bleeding, please go to the ER" in Spanish, you would say:

<u>"Si tiene algún sangrado grave, por favor vaya a la sala de emergencias."</u>

Here's the breakdown of the sentence:
"Si tiene" means "If you have," where "tiene" is the formal second person singular form of the verb "tener" (to have).
"algún sangrado grave" means "any severe bleeding."
"por favor" means "please"
"vaya" means "go," where "vaya" is the formal command form of the verb "ir" (to go).
"a la sala de emergencias" means "to the emergency room."

- To say "The risk of this procedure is pain, bleeding, infection" in Spanish, you would say:

<u>"El riesgo de este procedimiento es dolor, sangrado, infección."</u>

Here's the breakdown of the sentence:

"El riesgo de este procedimiento es" means "The risk of this procedure is."
"dolor" means "pain."
"sangrado" means "bleeding."
"infección" means "infection."

- To say "The ultrasound shows you have an ovarian cyst" in Spanish, you would say:

"el ultrasonido muestra que tiene un quiste ovárico."

Here's the breakdown of the sentence:
"el ultrasonido " means "The ultrasound."
"muestra" means "shows"
"que" means "that"
"tiene" means "you have."
"un quiste" means "a cyst"
"ovárico" means "ovarian."

- To say "I need to send you for more investigations" in Spanish, you would say:

"Necesito enviarlo/a para más investigaciones."

Here's the breakdown of the sentence:
"Necesito" means "I need."
"enviarlo/a" means "to send you," where "lo" is used for a male patient and "la" is used for a female patient.
"para" means "for"
"más" means "more"
"investigaciones" means "investigations."

-    To say "I need to order a blood test to determine whether it's malignant or benign" in Spanish, you would say:

"Necesito solicitar un análisis de sangre para determinar si es maligno o benigno."

Here's the breakdown of the sentence:
"Necesito" means "I need."
"solicitar" means "to order"
"un análisis de sangre" means "a blood test."
"para" means "for or to"
"determinar" means "determine"
"si" means "if or wehther"
"es maligno o benigno" means "it's malignant or benign."

-    To say "I need to send you for an MRI scan" in Spanish, you would say:

"Necesito enviarlo/a para una resonancia magnética."

Here's the breakdown of the sentence:
"Necesito" means "I need."
"enviarlo/a" means "to send you," where "lo" is used for a male patient and "la" is used for a female patient.
"para una resonancia magnética" means "for an MRI scan."

-       To say "The ovarian cyst you have is a simple cyst" in Spanish, you would say:

<u>"El quiste ovárico que tiene es un quiste simple."</u>

Here's the breakdown of the sentence:
"El quiste ovárico" means "The ovarian cyst."
"que tiene" means "you have."
"es un quiste simple" means "is a simple cyst."

-       To say "I need to book you for a repeat ultrasound in six to eight weeks to ensure its resolution" in Spanish, you would say:

<u>"Necesito programarle una repetición de el ultrasonido en seis a ocho semanas para asegurarnos de su resolución."</u>

Here's the breakdown of the sentence:
"Necesito programarle" means "I need to book you," where "programarle" is the formal way to say "book you" or "schedule for you."
"una repetición" means "a repeat"
"de el ultrasonido " means "of the ultrasound."
"en seis a ocho" means "in six to eight"
"semanas" means "weeks."
"para asegurarnos de su resolución" means "to ensure its resolution."

- To say "You don't need surgery for a simple cyst" in Spanish, you would say:

<u>"No necesita cirugía para un quiste simple."</u>

Here's the breakdown of the sentence:
"No necesita" means "You don't need."
"cirugía" means "surgery"
"para" means "for"
"un quiste simple" means "a simple cyst."

- To say "You need surgery to have the cyst removed" in Spanish, you would say:

<u>"Necesita cirugía para que le retiren el quiste."</u>

Here's the breakdown of the sentence:
"Necesita cirugía" means "You need surgery."
"para que le retiren" means "to have it removed for you,"
"el quiste" means "the cyst."

Acknowledgment

A heartfelt thank you to Vanessa Fuentes, whose invaluable assistance played an instrumental role in refining the language and enhancing the presentation of this book. Your keen eye for detail and dedication to ensuring that every word resonates with clarity and accuracy has made a substantial difference. Your support and expertise have not only enriched the content but have also helped in shaping this book into a more impactful resource for both healthcare professionals and the patients we aim to serve. Your collaborative spirit and commitment to excellence are deeply appreciated.

Other Books by OA Publications

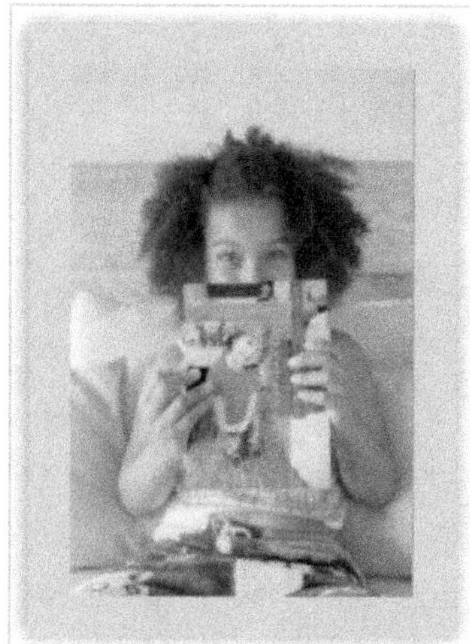

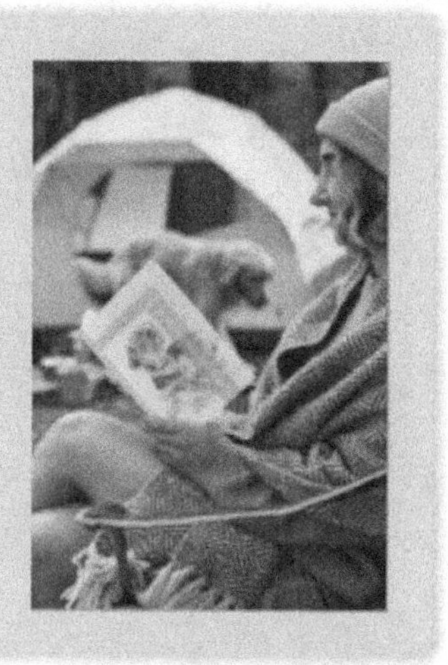

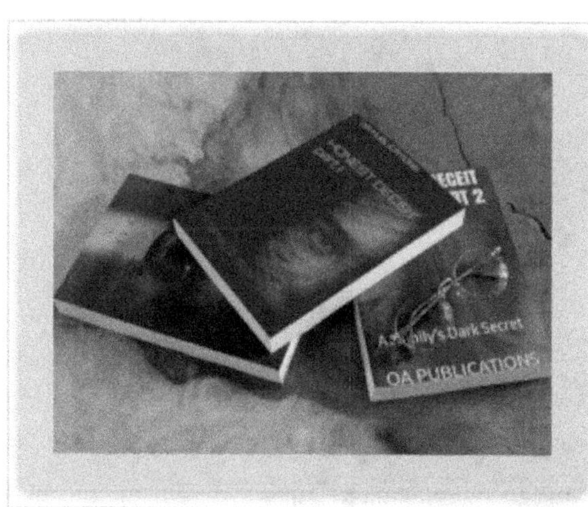

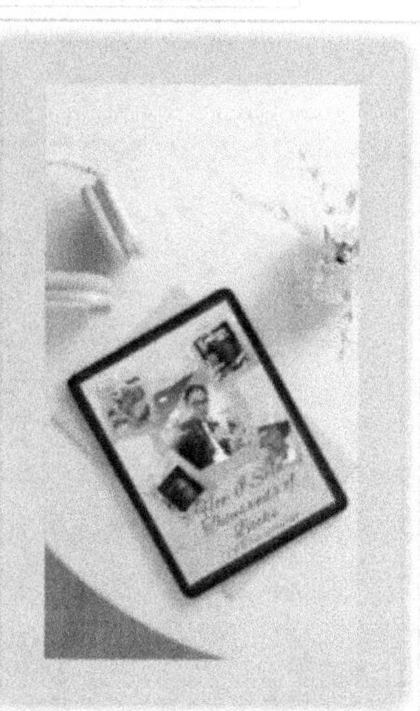

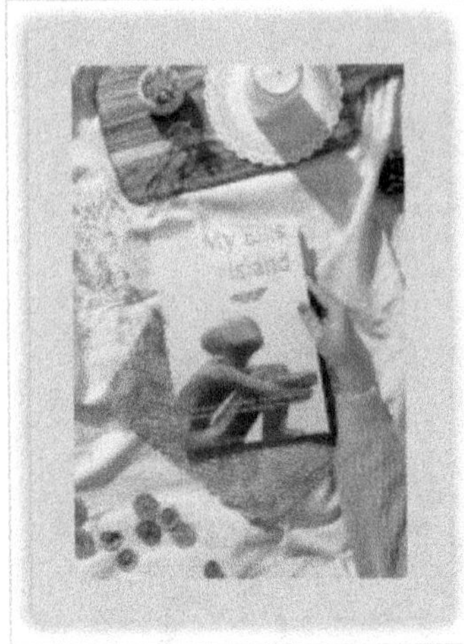

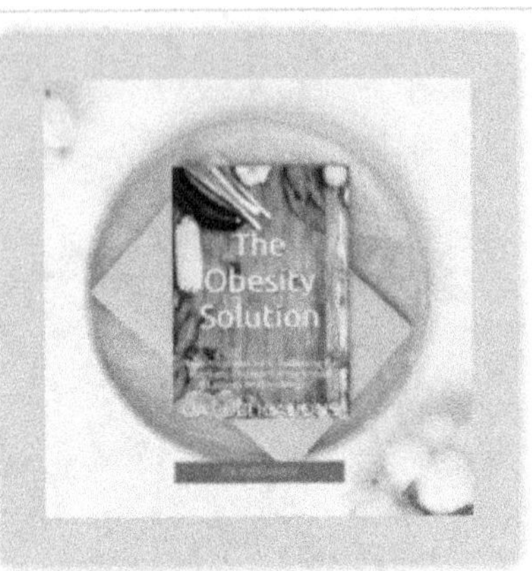

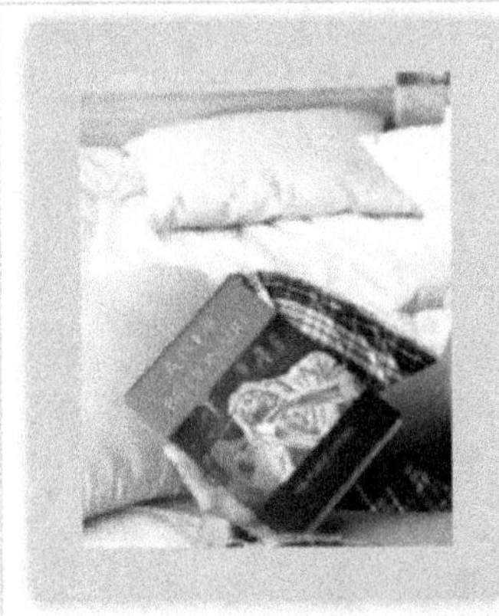

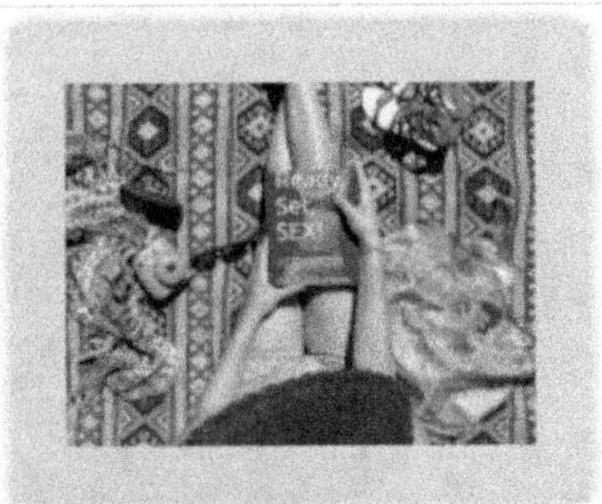

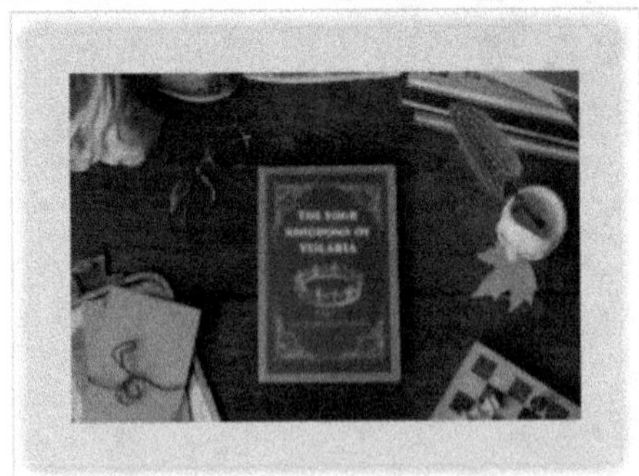